The Complete Dash Diet Cookbook 2021

- An Exhaustive Beginner's Cookbook to Lower Your Blood Pressure and Improve Your Health -

[Sebastian Osborne]

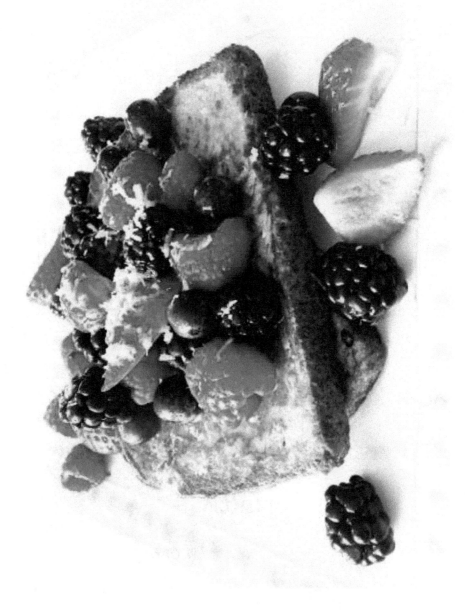

Table Of Content

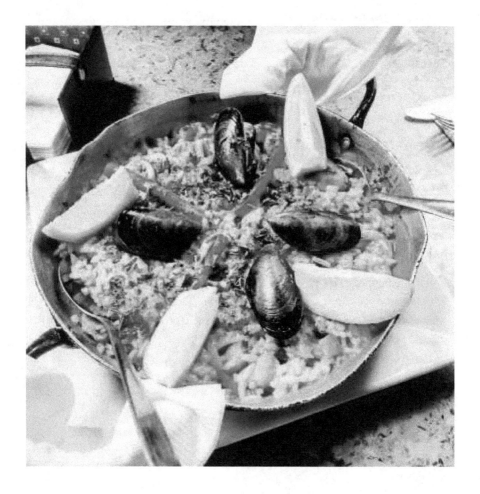

The following Book is reproduced below with the goal of providing information that is as accurate and reliable as possible. Regardless, purchasing this Book can be seen as consent to the fact that both the publisher and the author of this book are in no way experts on the topics discussed within and that any recommendations or suggestions that are made herein are for entertainment purposes only. Professionals should be consulted as needed prior to undertaking any of the action endorsed herein.

This declaration is deemed fair and valid by both the American Bar Association and the Committee of Publishers Association and is legally binding throughout the United States.

Furthermore, the transmission, duplication, or reproduction of any of the following work including specific information will be considered an illegal act irrespective of if it is done electronically or in print. This extends to creating a secondary or tertiary copy of the work or a recorded copy and is only allowed with the express written consent from the Publisher. All additional right reserved.

The information in the following pages is broadly considered a truthful and accurate account of facts and as such, any inattention, use, or misuse of the information in question by the reader will render any resulting actions solely under their purview. There are no scenarios in which the publisher or the original author of this work can be in any fashion deemed liable for any hardship or damages that may befall them after undertaking information described herein.

Additionally, the information in the following pages is intended only for informational purposes and should thus be thought of as universal. As befitting its nature, it is presented without assurance regarding its prolonged validity or interim quality. Trademarks that are mentioned are done without written consent and can in no way be considered an endorsement from the trademark holder.

CHAPTER 1: **BREAKFAST**

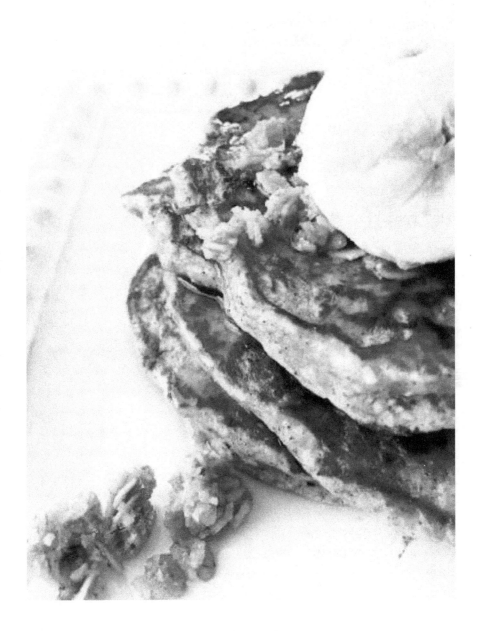

Banana Nut Pancakes

Prep:

15 mins

Cook:

4 mins

Total:

19 mins

Servings:

3

Yield:

6 to 8 pancakes

Ingredients

1 cup all-purpose flour

¼ cup finely chopped walnuts

1 tablespoon baking powder

½ teaspoon ground nutmeg

½ teaspoon ground cinnamon

3 tablespoons white sugar

½ teaspoon baking soda

½ teaspoon salt

2 small overripe bananas, mashed

1 ½ tablespoons butter, melted

1 cup almond milk

½ teaspoon vanilla extract

1 egg

Directions

1

Mix flour, walnuts, sugar, baking powder, nutmeg, cinnamon, baking soda, and salt in a large bowl; make a well in the center.

2

Whisk almond milk, bananas, melted butter, and vanilla extract together in a separate bowl until smooth. Whisk in egg. Pour mixture into the well in the flour mixture; stir until just combined.

3

Heat a lightly oiled skillet over medium-high heat. Drop 1/4 cup batter into the skillet; tilt gently to spread batter evenly. Cook until bubbles form and the edges are firm, 3 to 4 minutes. Flip and cook until browned on the other side, 1 to 3 minutes more. Repeat with remaining batter.

Nutrition

Per Serving: 427 calories; protein 9.1g; carbohydrates 65.5g; fat 15.5g; cholesterol 77.3mg; sodium 1052.4mg.

Breakfast Bread Pudding

Prep:

25 mins

Cook:

45 mins

Additional:

8 hrs 5 mins

Total:

9 hrs 15 mins

Servings:

12

Yield:

1 9x13-inch baking dish

Ingredients

6 eggs

1 cup milk

1 teaspoon ground cinnamon

½ cup heavy cream

1 tablespoon vanilla extract

1 (16 ounce) loaf cinnamon bread with raisins, cut into 1-inch cubes

2 Granny Smith apples - peeled, cored, and sliced

1 teaspoon ground nutmeg

1 cup brown sugar

¼ cup melted butter

1 Granny Smith apple - peeled, cored, and diced

Directions

1

Beat the eggs in a mixing bowl. Whisk in the milk, cream, vanilla extract, and nutmeg until evenly blended. Fold in the bread cubes and set aside until the bread soaks up the egg mixture, about 5 minutes. Place the sliced apples into a mixing bowl and sprinkle with brown sugar, cinnamon, and melted butter; toss to evenly coat. Grease a 9x13-inch baking dish and arrange the apple slices evenly into the bottom of the prepared baking dish; spoon the bread mixture over top. Cover the dish with aluminum foil and refrigerate overnight.

2

Preheat an oven to 375 degrees F.

3

Sprinkle the diced apple over the bread pudding and cover again with the aluminum foil. Bake in the preheated oven until the bread is no longer soggy, about 40 minutes. Remove the foil and set the oven to Broil; broil until golden brown on top, about 5-6 minutes. Remove and let stand 5 to 10 minutes before serving.

Nutrition

Per Serving: 312 calories; protein 8.3g; carbohydrates 43g; fat 12.5g; cholesterol 118.4mg; sodium 221.7mg.

Orange-Blueberry Muffin

Prep:

25 mins

Cook:

15 mins

Additional:

20 mins

Total:

1 hr

Servings:

12

Yield:

12 muffins

Ingredients

½ cup oat bran
1 cup wheat bran
½ cup sour cream
1 cup all-purpose flour
1 teaspoon baking powder
1 teaspoon baking soda
½ cup milk
⅔ cup brown sugar
½ teaspoon salt
⅓ cup vegetable oil
1 orange, juiced and zested
1 cup fresh blueberries
1 egg
1 teaspoon vanilla extract

Directions

1

Preheat an oven to 375 degrees F. Grease 12 muffin cups, or line with paper muffin liners.

2

Combine the oat bran and wheat bran in a large bowl. Stir in sour cream and milk. Allow mixture to stand for 10 minutes. Combine flour, baking powder, baking soda, brown sugar, and salt in a separate bowl. Gently stir blueberries into the flour mixture, carefully coating all the blueberries with flour. Stir vegetable oil, orange juice and zest, egg, and vanilla extract into the bran mixture. Combine flour mixture with the wet **Ingredients** until just blended. Drop batter into lined muffin cups.

3

Bake in the preheated oven until a toothpick inserted into the center comes out clean, 15 to 20 minutes. Cool in the pans for 10 minutes before removing to cool completely on a wire rack.

Nutrition

Per Serving: 182 calories; protein 3.8g; carbohydrates 24.4g; fat 9.3g; cholesterol 20.5mg; sodium 260.4mg.

Spiced Oatmeal

Prep:

5 mins

Cook:

2 mins

Total:

7 mins

Servings:

1

Yield:

1 serving

Ingredients

¾ cup old-fashioned rolled oats

½ cup frozen blueberries

1 cup water

¼ cup orange juice

½ teaspoon ground cinnamon

¼ cup dried cranberries

Directions

1

Place the rolled oats, cinnamon, cranberries, and blueberries in a microwave safe bowl. Add the turmeric and ginger, if desired. Pour in the water, and stir to mix **Ingredients**. Cook on High until water is absorbed, about 2 minutes. Stir in orange juice to desired consistency.

Nutrition

Per Serving: 398 calories; protein 9.1g; carbohydrates 84.8g; fat 4.5g; sodium 12.7mg.

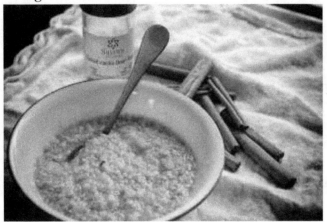

Creamy Mushroom Grits

Prep:

10 mins

Cook:

45 mins

Additional:

8 hrs 30 mins

Total:

9 hrs 25 mins

Servings:

4

Yield:

4 large servings

Ingredients

1 cup stone-ground white corn grits

½ cup shredded Parmesan cheese

4 dried morel mushrooms, or more to taste

3 cups whole milk

3 cups vegetarian chicken-flavored broth

Directions

1

Place grits in a bowl with water to cover. Set aside to soak, 8 hours to overnight. Skim any debris that floats to top, rinse well, and drain.

2

Bring broth to a boil in a saucepan; remove from heat. Add mushrooms and soak until soft, about 30 minutes. Strain mushrooms, reserving broth. Chop mushrooms.

3

Bring reserved broth and milk to a boil in saucepan over high heat. Stir grits in gradually, add mushrooms, and decrease heat to low. Cover and cook, stirring occasionally, until grits are soft and creamy, 40 to 50 minutes. Stir in Parmesan cheese until melted.

Nutrition

Per Serving: 310 calories; protein 14.3g; carbohydrates 41.9g; fat 9.3g; cholesterol 27.1mg; sodium 564mg.

Veggies Bakes

Prep:

20 mins

Cook:

40 mins

Total:

1 hr

Servings:

4

Yield:

4 servings

Ingredients

2 large red onions, each cut into 8 wedges

2 large carrots, cut into 1/2-inch slices

½ teaspoon ground cumin

½ large rutabaga, peeled and cut into 3/4-inch cubes

½ cup olive oil

3 tablespoons butter, melted

1 ½ teaspoons curry powder

1 ½ large sweet potatoes, cut into 3/4-inch slices, then into thirds

¾ teaspoon ground turmeric

½ teaspoon salt

Directions

1

Preheat oven to 450 degrees F.

2

Combine red onions, carrots, sweet potatoes, and rutabaga in a large bowl. Pour in olive oil and butter. Add curry powder, turmeric, salt, and cumin; toss until thoroughly coated. Transfer to a large baking dish.

3

Bake in the preheated oven, uncovered, until almost tender, 20 to 30 minutes. Toss. Continue baking until vegetables are fork-tender, 20 to 30 minutes more.

Nutrition
Per Serving: 546 calories; protein 5.3g; carbohydrates 53.4g; fat 36.3g; cholesterol 22.9mg; sodium 494.3mg.

Honey Lime Fruit Toss

Prep:

10 mins

Total:

10 mins

Servings:

7

Yield:

7 servings

Ingredients

1 (20 ounce) can DOLE® Pineapple Chunks

1 DOLE Banana, sliced

1 DOLE Kiwi Fruit, peeled, halved, sliced

1 cup quartered DOLE Fresh or Frozen Strawberries

¼ teaspoon grated lime peel

1 (11 ounce) can DOLE Mandarin Oranges, drained

1 tablespoon honey

2 tablespoons fresh lime juice

Directions

1

Drain pineapple; reserve 1/4 cup juice.

2

Combine pineapple chunks, mandarin oranges, banana, kiwi fruit and strawberries in large serving bowl.

3

Stir together reserved pineapple juice, lime peel, lime juice and honey in small bowl. Pour over salad; toss to coat.

Nutrition

Per Serving: 110 calories; protein 0.4g; carbohydrates 27.3g; fat 0.1g; sodium 10.5mg.

Egg Muffins

Prep:

10 mins

Cook:

20 mins

Total:

30 mins

Servings:

12

Yield:

12 servings

Ingredients

½ pound bulk pork sausage

12 eggs

½ cup chopped green bell pepper, or to taste

½ teaspoon salt

¼ teaspoon ground black pepper

½ cup chopped onion

½ cup shredded Cheddar cheese

¼ teaspoon garlic powder

Directions

1

Preheat oven to 350 degrees F. Lightly grease 12 muffin cups, or line with paper muffin liners.

2

Heat a large skillet over medium-high heat and stir in sausage; cook and stir until sausage is crumbly, evenly browned, and no longer pink, 10 to 15 minutes; drain.

3

Beat eggs in a large bowl. Stir in onion, green pepper, salt, pepper, and garlic powder. Mix in sausage and Cheddar cheese. Spoon by 1/3 cupfuls into muffin cups.

4

Bake in preheated oven until a knife inserted near the center comes out clean, 20 to 23 minutes.

Nutrition

Per Serving: 143 calories; protein 10.2g; carbohydrates 1.6g; fat 10.6g; cholesterol 201.7mg; sodium 364.8mg.

Hearty Porridge

Prep:

10 mins

Cook:

15 mins

Total:

25 mins

Servings:

7

Yield:

7 servings

Ingredients

1 cup rolled oats

2 tablespoons ground cinnamon

½ cup quinoa

½ cup raisins

½ cup almond meal

½ cup flaxseed meal

½ cup chopped walnuts

1 small apple, chopped

3 ½ cups water

½ cup shredded coconut

Directions

1

Combine oats, quinoa, raisins, walnuts, almond meal, flaxseed meal, coconut, apple, and cinnamon in a pot; add water. Bring mixture to a boil, stirring regularly; reduce heat and simmer until oats are tender and liquid is absorbed, about 9 minutes.

Nutrition

Per Serving: 319 calories; protein 8.6g; carbohydrates 34.2g; fat 18.7g; sodium 14.2mg.

Millet Cream

Prep:

5 mins

Cook:

25 mins

Total:

30 mins

Servings:

4

Yield:

4 servings

Ingredients

3 cups water

1 cup millet

¼ teaspoon salt

Directions

1

Bring water to a boil in a pot. Add millet and salt. Return to a boil, stirring frequently. Cover and let simmer over medium-low heat until water is absorbed and millet is fluffy, about 15-17 minutes.

Nutrition

Per Serving: 189 calories; protein 5.5g; carbohydrates 36.4g; fat 2.1g; sodium 153.2mg.

Vanilla Toast

Prep:

10 mins

Cook:

10 mins

Total:

20 mins

Servings:

4

Yield:

8 slices

Ingredients

2 cups whole milk

4 large eggs

½ teaspoon almond extract (such as Watkins® pure almond extract)

½ teaspoon ground cinnamon

¼ teaspoon ground nutmeg

1 teaspoon double-strength imitation vanilla extract (such as Goodman's Route 66)

2 tablespoons brown sugar

8 thick slices slightly stale Texas toast

⅛ teaspoon ground allspice

Directions

1

Mix whole milk and brown sugar in a large bowl.

2

Beat eggs, vanilla extract, almond extract, cinnamon, nutmeg, and allspice together in a separate bowl until the eggs are well beaten; add to the milk mixture and stir to dissolve the brown sugar.

3

Heat a non-stick skillet or griddle over medium-low heat.

4

Set one slice of Texas toast into the milk mixture; let soak until moistened, about 12 seconds per side.

5

Cook the dipped toast in the preheated skillet until bottom is golden brown, 3 to 5 minutes; flip toast and continue to cook until the other side is browned, 4 - 6 minutes more. Repeat dipping and cooking with remaining bread slices.

Nutrition

Per Serving: 337 calories; protein 14.8g; carbohydrates 43.4g; fat 11g; cholesterol 198.2mg; sodium 529.5mg.

Cherry Rice

Prep:

10 mins

Cook:

1 hr 1 min

Total:

1 hr 11 mins

Servings:

4

Yield:

4 servings

Ingredients

2 ½ cups water, divided

½ cup wild rice

2 tablespoons red wine vinegar

¼ cup brown rice

½ cup brown sugar

¼ cup sliced almonds

½ cup sliced celery

⅓ cup fresh orange juice

1 cup pitted and sliced cherries

1 teaspoon grated orange zest

Directions

1

Bring 2 cups water and wild rice to a boil in a saucepan. Reduce heat to medium-low, cover, and simmer until rice is tender, 30 to 45 minutes. Drain excess liquid, fluff rice with a fork, and cook uncovered, about 5-7 minutes more.

2

Bring 1/2 water and brown rice to a boil in a saucepan. Reduce heat to medium-low, cover, and simmer until rice is tender and liquid has been absorbed, about 45-50 minutes.

3

Combine cherries, brown sugar, and almonds in a large nonstick skillet; cook and stir over medium heat until brown sugar melts and coats cherries and almonds, about 5 minutes. Stir in brown rice, wild rice, celery, orange juice, red wine vinegar, and orange zest. Cook, stirring frequently, until heated through, about 5 minutes.

Nutrition

Per Serving: 295 calories; protein 5.8g; carbohydrates 61.4g; fat 3.9g; sodium 26.2mg.

CHAPTER 2: LUNCH

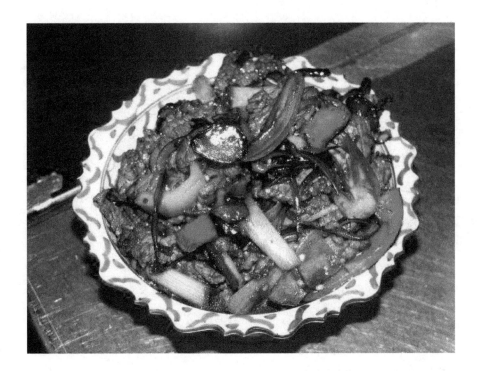

Thai Steak

Prep:

15 mins

Cook:

10 mins

Total:

25 mins

Servings:

6

Yield:

6 servings

Ingredients

½ teaspoon ground black pepper

¼ teaspoon kosher salt

¼ cup fresh lime juice

2 tablespoons soy sauce

1 tablespoon brown sugar

⅓ cup fresh Thai basil leaves

1 tablespoon fish sauce

1 (1 1/2-pound) flank steak

2 teaspoons minced garlic

2 heads romaine lettuce

⅓ cup fresh mint leaves

⅓ cup fresh cilantro leaves

1 teaspoon chile-garlic sauce (such as Sriracha®)

Directions

1

Preheat an outdoor grill for medium-high heat and lightly oil the grate. Sprinkle pepper and salt onto flank steak.

2

Cook steak on preheated grill until desired doneness is reached, 5 to 6 minutes per side. An instant-read thermometer inserted into the center should read 140 degrees F.

3

Whisk lime juice, soy sauce, brown sugar, fish sauce, garlic, and chile-garlic sauce together in a bowl.

4

Mix romaine lettuce, mint, cilantro, and basil together in a bowl; spoon about 6 tablespoons lime juice mixture over romaine mixture. Toss to coat.

5

Cut steak into strips and place strips into remaining lime juice mixture; let sit for steak to marinate, approximately 2 minutes. Place steak on romaine mixture.

Nutrition

Per Serving: 132 calories; protein 15.7g; carbohydrates 8g; fat 4.5g; cholesterol 26.9mg; sodium 639.5mg.

Hoisin Pork

Prep:

30 mins

Cook:

20 mins

Total:

50 mins

Servings:

4

Yield:

4 servings

Ingredients

1 pound boneless pork chops, cut into stir-fry strips

1 tablespoon hoisin sauce

1 tablespoon cornstarch

2 tablespoons hoisin sauce

1 tablespoon white sugar

1 teaspoon red pepper flakes, or to taste

1 tablespoon sesame oil

2 cloves garlic, minced

¼ cup chicken broth

2 teaspoons minced fresh ginger root

1 tablespoon cornstarch

1 tablespoon rice vinegar

1 carrot, peeled and sliced

1 (4 ounce) can sliced water chestnuts, drained

2 green onions, sliced

1 green bell pepper, sliced

Directions

1

Mix the sliced pork, 1 tablespoon hoisin sauce, and 1 tablespoon cornstarch together in a bowl. Set aside. Combine the remaining 2 tablespoons hoisin sauce, chicken broth, and 1 tablespoon cornstarch with rice vinegar, sugar, and cayenne pepper in small bowl. Set aside.

2

Heat the sesame oil in a skillet over medium-high heat. Stir in the pork; cook and stir until the pork begins to brown, about 5 minutes. Add the garlic and ginger; cook and stir until fragrant. Mix in the carrot, bell pepper, and water chestnuts, cooking until the carrots are tender. Stir in the reserved hoisin sauce mixture and continue cooking and stirring until the flavors are combined, about 3 minutes.

Nutrition

Per Serving: 235 calories; protein 15.6g; carbohydrates 17.5g; fat 11.4g; cholesterol 39.3mg; sodium 295.2mg.

Tomato Bean Soup

Prep:

15 mins

Cook:

30 mins

Total:

45 mins

Servings:

4

Yield:

4 servings

Ingredients

1 (15 ounce) can black beans, undrained

1 cup low-sodium chicken broth

cooking spray

1 (15 ounce) can black beans, undrained

1 small onion, chopped

2 teaspoons ground cumin

1 teaspoon minced garlic

1 (10 ounce) can diced tomatoes with green chile peppers (such as RO*TEL®)

4 teaspoons lime juice

2 tablespoons chopped fresh cilantro

Directions

1

Place 1 can black beans and chicken broth into a blender. Cover and puree until smooth.

2

Heat a large saucepan coated with cooking spray over medium-high heat; cook and stir onion and garlic until onion is tender, about 5 minutes. Stir remaining 1 can black beans and liquid, tomatoes, yogurt, lime juice, cumin, red pepper flakes, and pureed beans into onion mixture; bring to a boil. Reduce heat to low, cover, and simmer for 25 to 30 minutes, stirring occasionally. Garnish with cilantro to serve.

Nutrition

Per Serving: 237 calories; protein 15.7g; carbohydrates 42.3g; fat 1.5g; cholesterol 2.2mg; sodium 1142.6mg.

Paella

Prep:

30 mins

Cook:

30 mins

Total:

1 hr

Servings:

8

Yield:

8 servings

Ingredients

2 tablespoons olive oil

1 tablespoon paprika

2 pounds skinless, boneless chicken breasts, cut into 2 inch pieces

2 tablespoons olive oil, divided

3 cloves garlic, crushed

2 teaspoons dried oregano

1 teaspoon crushed red pepper flakes

1 pinch saffron threads

salt and black pepper to taste

1 bay leaf

1 quart chicken stock

2 lemons, zested

2 tablespoons olive oil

½ bunch Italian flat leaf parsley, chopped

1 Spanish onion, chopped

1 red bell pepper, coarsely chopped

1 pound chorizo sausage, casings removed and crumbled

2 cups uncooked short-grain white rice

1 pound shrimp, peeled and deveined

Directions

1

In a medium bowl, mix together 2 tablespoons olive oil, paprika, oregano, and salt and pepper. Stir in chicken pieces to coat. Cover, and refrigerate.

2

Heat 2 tablespoons olive oil in a large skillet or paella pan over medium heat. Stir in garlic, red pepper flakes, and rice. Cook, stirring, to coat rice with oil, about 3 minutes. Stir in saffron threads, bay leaf, parsley, chicken stock, and lemon zest. Bring to a boil, cover, and reduce heat to medium low. Simmer 20 minutes.

3

Meanwhile, heat 2 tablespoons olive oil in a separate skillet over medium heat. Stir in marinated chicken and onion; cook 5 minutes. Stir in bell pepper and sausage; cook 5 minutes. Stir in shrimp; cook, turning the shrimp, until both sides are pink.

4

Spread rice mixture onto a serving tray. Top with meat and seafood mixture.

Nutrition

Per Serving: 736 calories; protein 55.7g; carbohydrates 45.7g; fat 35.1g; cholesterol 202.5mg; sodium 1204.2mg.

Lime Calamari

Prep:

15 mins

Cook:

5 mins

Total:

20 mins

Servings:

10

Yield:

10 appetizer servings

Ingredients

3 cups vegetable oil

1 lemon - cut into wedges, for garnish

1 teaspoon salt

1 teaspoon dried oregano

½ teaspoon ground black pepper

12 squid, cleaned and sliced into rings

¼ cup all-purpose flour

Directions

1

Preheat oil in a heavy, deep frying pan or pot. Oil should be heated to 365 degrees F.

2

In a medium size mixing bowl mix together flour, salt, oregano and black pepper. Dredge squid through flour and spice mixture.

3

Place squid in oil for 2 to 3 minutes or until light brown. Beware of overcooking, squid will be tough if overcooked. Dry squid on paper towels. Serve with wedges of lemon.

Nutrition

Per Serving: 642 calories; protein 8g; carbohydrates 5.2g; fat 66.7g; cholesterol 111.8mg; sodium 254.1mg.

Sunshine Toast

Prep:

5 mins

Cook:

10 mins

Total:

15 mins

Servings:

1

Yield:

1 serving

Ingredients

1 egg
salt to taste
1 slice bread
2 tablespoons butter, divided

Directions

1

Melt 1 tablespoon butter in a small skillet over medium heat.

2

Using a glass or cookie cutter, create a hole in the middle of the bread, removing the center so it is perfectly circular. Butter the bread lightly on both sides and lightly fry it on one side, and then turn it over. Crack the egg into the hole in the middle of the bread and fry quickly. Be careful that the bread does not burn. Serve warm.

Nutrition

Per Serving: 342 calories; protein 8.4g; carbohydrates 13.1g; fat 28.8g; cholesterol 247.1mg; sodium 403.8mg

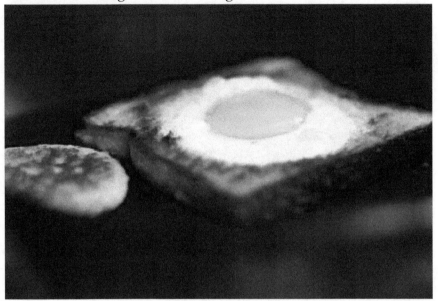

Chicken Noodle Soup

Prep:

20 mins

Cook:

1 hr

Total:

1 hr 20 mins

Servings:

12

Yield:

12 servings

Ingredients

3 tablespoons vegetable oil

6 carrot, diced

¾ tablespoon chopped fresh rosemary

¾ tablespoon chopped fresh tarragon

¾ tablespoon chopped fresh thyme

6 stalks celery, diced

¾ tablespoon chopped Italian flat leaf parsley

3 ½ cups cubed skinless, boneless chicken breast meat

1 (16 ounce) package egg noodles

4 quarts low-fat, low sodium chicken broth

salt and pepper to taste

2 onions, diced

Directions

1

In a large skillet over medium heat, cook onions in oil until translucent. Stir in celery, carrot, rosemary, tarragon, thyme and parsley and cook, covered, until vegetables are soft, 5 to 10 minutes.

2

Transfer vegetable mixture to a large pot and pour in chicken broth. Simmer over low heat, covered, for 30 minutes.

3

Stir in chicken breast pieces and egg noodles and simmer, covered, 30 minutes more. Season with salt and pepper.

Nutrition

Per Serving: 276 calories; protein 23.2g; carbohydrates 29.9g; fat 6.6g; cholesterol 65mg; sodium 593mg.

Banana Nut Muffins

Prep:

15 mins

Cook:

25 mins

Total:

40 mins

Servings:

18

Yield:

18 muffins

Ingredients

2 cups whole wheat pastry flour

¾ teaspoon baking soda

¾ teaspoon ground cinnamon

¼ teaspoon freshly ground nutmeg

1 cup finely chopped walnuts

¾ teaspoon salt

4 large ripe bananas

1 cup turbinado sugar

¼ cup canola oil

1 tablespoon vanilla extract

1 teaspoon apple cider vinegar

½ cup unsweetened almond milk

Directions

1

Preheat the oven to 375 degrees F. Line 18 muffin cups with liners.

2

Sift flour, baking soda, salt, cinnamon, and nutmeg together in a large bowl. Stir in walnuts and oats.

3

Combine bananas, sugar, almond milk, canola oil, vanilla extract, and vinegar in a separate bowl. Blend together until smooth. Add to the flour mixture. Stir until just combined.

4

Drop batter into the muffin cups, filling each completely full.

5

Bake in the preheated oven until a toothpick inserted into the center comes out clean, about 23 minutes. Transfer to a wire rack to cool.

Nutrition

Per Serving: 192 calories; protein 3.1g; carbohydrates 28.8g; fat 7.9g; sodium 158.7mg.

Kabobs

Prep:

30 mins

Cook:

10 mins

Additional:

4 hrs

Total:

4 hrs 40 mins

Servings:

10

Yield:

10 servings

Ingredients

½ cup teriyaki sauce
½ cup honey
½ teaspoon garlic powder
½ pinch ground ginger
2 red bell peppers, cut into 2 inch pieces
1 ½ cups whole fresh mushrooms
1 pound beef sirloin, cut into 1 inch cubes
1 ½ pounds skinless, boneless chicken breast halves - cut into cubes
Skewers
1 large sweet onion, peeled and cut into wedges

Directions

1

In a large resealable plastic bag, mix the teriyaki sauce, honey, garlic powder, and ginger. Place red bell peppers, onion wedges, mushrooms, beef, and chicken in the bag with the marinade. Seal, and refrigerate 4 to 24 hours.

2
Preheat grill for medium-high heat.

3
Discard marinade, and thread the meat and vegetables onto skewers, leaving a small space between each item.

4
Lightly oil the grill grate. Grill skewers for 10 minutes, turning as needed, or until meat is cooked through and vegetables are tender.

Nutrition
Per Serving: 304 calories; protein 24.8g; carbohydrates 21.2g; fat 13.3g; cholesterol 73.9mg; sodium 622.5mg.

Fish Tacos

Prep:

20 mins

Cook:

10 mins

Additional:

20 mins

Total:

50 mins

Servings:

8

Yield:

8 tacos

Ingredients

1 lime, juiced
1 jalapeno pepper, diced
¼ cup olive oil
¼ cup chopped cilantro
¼ teaspoon ground cumin
salt and ground black pepper to taste
½ pound halibut fillets
8 corn tortillas
1 tablespoon ground ancho chile powder
Toppings:
2 cups shredded cabbage
1 cup shredded pepper Jack cheese
1 avocado, sliced
1 (8 ounce) jar salsa

Directions

1

Stir lime juice, olive oil, cilantro, jalapeno, chile powder, cumin, salt, and pepper together in a large bowl or resealable zip-top bag. Add halibut and marinate for 20 to 25 minutes. Do not over-marinate, as lime juice will start to 'cook' the fish.

2

Preheat an outdoor grill for medium heat and lightly oil the grate. Drain marinade; grill fillets for 5 minutes. Turn and cook until fish flakes easily with a fork, about 2 minutes more.

3

Warm tortillas on the grill or stove. Divide halibut among tortillas and top with cabbage, salsa, pepper Jack cheese, and avocado.

Nutrition

Per Serving: 269 calories; protein 12.4g; carbohydrates 18.2g; fat 17.1g; cholesterol 28.2mg; sodium 321.1mg.

Roasted Cauliflower

Prep:

15 mins

Cook:

30 mins

Total:

45 mins

Servings:

4

Yield:

4 servings

Ingredients

1 large head cauliflower, cut into florets

2 tablespoons hoisin sauce

1 tablespoon Sriracha sauce

salt and ground black pepper to taste

2 tablespoons olive oil

Directions

1

Preheat the oven to 400 degrees F.

2

Combine cauliflower florets, olive oil, hoisin sauce, Sriracha sauce, salt, and pepper in a large bowl; toss to combine. Spread out in a single layer on a baking sheet.

3

Bake in the preheated oven until cauliflower is soft and cooked through, about 30 minutes, turning once after 20 minutes.

Nutrition

Per Serving: 132 calories; protein 4.4g; carbohydrates 15g; fat 7.2g; cholesterol 0.2mg; sodium 389.8mg.

Blackened Tuna

Prep:

10 mins

Cook:

10 mins

Total:

20 mins

Servings:

6

Yield:

6 servings

Ingredients

1 ½ pounds fresh tuna steaks, 1 inch thick

2 tablespoons olive oil

2 tablespoons butter

2 tablespoons Cajun seasoning

Directions

1

Generously coat tuna with Cajun seasoning.

2

Heat oil and butter in a large skillet over high heat. When oil is nearly smoking, place steaks in pan. Cook on one side for 4 minutes, or until blackened. Turn steaks, and cook for 3 to 4 minutes.

Nutrition

Per Serving: 243 calories; protein 26.7g; carbohydrates 1.1g; fat 14g; cholesterol 53.5mg; sodium 545.6mg.

CHAPTER 3: DINNER

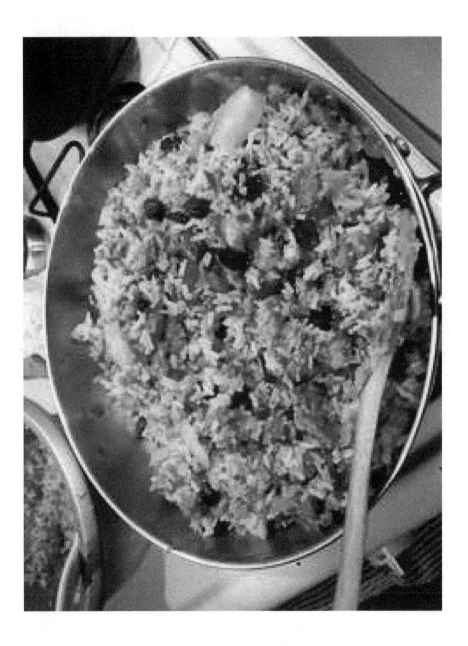

Brown Rice Pilaf

Prep:

10 mins

Cook:

55 mins

Total:

1 hr 5 mins

Servings:

2

Yield:

2 servings

Ingredients

½ cup fresh corn kernels

½ cup brown rice

1 ¼ cups chicken broth

½ cup chopped onion

1 tablespoon olive oil

Directions

1

Heat olive oil in a small saucepan over medium heat. Add corn and onion; cook and stir until lightly browned, 5 to 7 minutes. Add rice and stir to coat with oil. Add chicken broth and bring to a boil. Cover and reduce heat to low. Cook until rice is tender, about 45 minutes.

Nutrition

Per Serving: 259 calories; protein 4.8g; carbohydrates 40.7g; fat 8.4g; cholesterol 3.8mg; sodium 730.9mg.

Pantry Puttanesca

Prep:

5 mins

Cook:

16 mins

Total:

21 mins

Servings:

4

Yield:

4 servings

Ingredients

⅓ cup olive oil

¼ cup capers, chopped

3 cloves garlic, minced

¼ teaspoon crushed red pepper flakes

1 teaspoon dried oregano

2 (15 ounce) cans diced tomatoes, drained.

1 (8 ounce) package spaghetti

½ cup chopped pitted kalamata olives

3 anchovy fillets, chopped

Directions

1

Fill a large pot with water. Bring to a rolling boil over high heat.

2

As the water heats, pour the olive oil into a cold skillet and stir in the garlic. Turn heat to medium-low and cook and stir until the garlic is fragrant and begins to turn a golden color, 1 to 2 minutes. Stir in the red pepper flakes, oregano, and anchovies. Cook until anchovies begin to break down, about 2 minutes.

3

Pour tomatoes into skillet, turn heat to medium-high, and bring sauce to a simmer. Use the back of a spoon to break down tomatoes as they cook. Simmer until sauce is reduced and combined, about 12 minutes.

4

Meanwhile, cook the pasta in the boiling water. Drain when still very firm to the bite, about 10 minutes. Reserve 1/2 cup pasta water.

5

Stir the olives and capers into the sauce; add pasta and toss to combine.

6

Toss pasta in sauce until pasta is cooked through and well coated with sauce, about 1 minute. If sauce becomes too thick, stir in some of the reserved pasta water to thin.

Nutrition

Per Serving: 463 calories; protein 10.5g; carbohydrates 53.3g; fat 24g; cholesterol 2.5mg; sodium 944.5mg.

Cinnamon Toast

Prep:

5 mins

Cook:

2 mins

Total:

7 mins

Servings:

2

Yield:

2 servings

Ingredients

2 slices white bread
2 teaspoons butter or margarine
1 teaspoon ground cinnamon
2 tablespoons white sugar

Directions

1

Use a toaster to toast the bread to desired darkness. Spread butter or margarine onto one side of each slice. In a cup or small bowl, stir together the sugar and cinnamon; sprinkle generously over hot buttered toast.

Nutrition

Per Serving: 154 calories; protein 2g; carbohydrates 26.1g; fat 4.9g; cholesterol 10.8mg; sodium 199.2mg.

Polenta with Vegetables

Prep:

30 mins

Cook:

30 mins

Total:

1 hr

Servings:

6

Yield:

6 servings

Ingredients

1 (16 ounce) tube polenta, cut into 1/2 inch slices

1 (16 ounce) can black beans

1 (10 ounce) can whole kernel corn

⅓ cup black olives

1 onion, chopped

1 green bell pepper, chopped

1 (15 ounce) can kidney beans

1 small eggplant, peeled and cubed

1 (1.27 ounce) packet dry fajita seasoning

1 (8 ounce) jar salsa

1 cup shredded mozzarella cheese

6 fresh mushrooms, chopped

Directions

1

Preheat oven to 350 degrees F. Lightly oil a 9x13 inch baking dish.

2

Heat oil in a skillet over medium heat. Cook and stir onion, green pepper, eggplant, and mushrooms in oil until soft. Mix in fajita seasoning.

3

Line prepared baking dish with slices of polenta. Spread beans and corn evenly over the polenta, and then spread onion mixture over the beans. Top with salsa, mozzarella cheese and black olives.

4

Bake until heated through, about 20 minutes.

Nutrition

Per Serving: 329 calories; protein 17.8g; carbohydrates 57.5g; fat 5g; cholesterol 12.1mg; sodium 1633.4mg.

Herbed Sole

Prep:

15 mins

Cook:

30 mins

Total:

45 mins

Servings:

4

Yield:

4 servings

Ingredients

1 tablespoon lemon juice
1 tablespoon all-purpose flour
2 tablespoons thinly sliced green onion
1 clove garlic, minced
¼ cup dry white wine
4 (6 ounce) fillets sole
salt to taste
ground black pepper to taste
¼ teaspoon paprika
¼ pound cooked salad shrimp
2 tablespoons butter

Directions

1

In a small bowl, combine lemon juice, green onion, garlic, and wine. Set aside.

2

Lay filets flat, and divide shrimp evenly among them in a band across one end of each fillet. Roll up around shrimp, and secure with toothpick. Place in a baking dish. Season to taste with salt, pepper, and paprika. Pour lemon juice mixture over the fish. Cover.

3

Bake at 350 degrees F for 25 minutes.

4

When fillets are nearly done, prepare sauce. In a small saucepan, melt butter over medium heat. Stir in flour. Transfer fish to serving platter ,and keep warm. Pour pan juices into butter/flour mixture; cook and stir until thickened. Pour over sole, and serve.

Nutrition

Per Serving: 253 calories; protein 37.5g; carbohydrates 2.8g; fat 8.1g; cholesterol 149.9mg; sodium 226.5mg.

Cucumber Salad

Prep:

15 mins

Additional:

20 mins

Total:

35 mins

Servings:

8

Yield:

8 servings

Ingredients

2 large cucumbers, peeled and sliced

2 tablespoons white vinegar

1 ½ tablespoons sour cream

1 teaspoon salt

½ cup diced sweet onion (such as Vidalia®)

½ teaspoon cracked black pepper

2 tablespoons white sugar

Directions

1

Combine cucumbers, onion, vinegar, sugar, sour cream, salt, and pepper together in a bowl.

2

Cover bowl with plastic wrap and refrigerate until chilled, 20 to 30 minutes.

Nutrition

Per Serving: 31 calories; protein 0.6g; carbohydrates 6.1g; fat 0.7g; cholesterol 1.2mg; sodium 294mg.

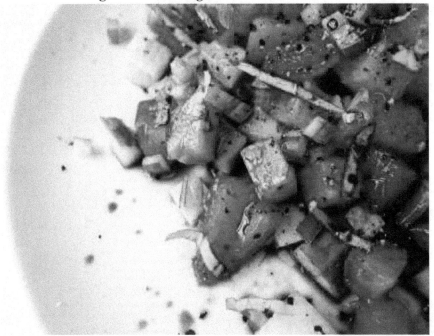

Golden Eggplant Fries

Prep:

15 mins

Cook:

15 mins

Additional:

5 mins

Total:

35 mins

Servings:

4

Yield:

4 servings

Ingredients

1 medium eggplant

½ cup Italian bread crumbs

1 teaspoon Italian seasoning

1 teaspoon salt

½ teaspoon dried basil

¼ cup freshly grated Parmesan cheese

½ teaspoon garlic powder

½ teaspoon ground black pepper

¼ cup all-purpose flour

2 eggs

½ teaspoon onion powder

Directions

1

Slice eggplant into 1/2-inch rounds, then cut each round into 1/4-inch sticks. Pat dry.

2

Combine bread crumbs, Parmesan cheese, Italian seasoning, salt, basil, garlic powder, onion powder, and black pepper in a shallow bowl. Pour flour into a second shallow bowl. Beat eggs in a third bowl.

3

Dip eggplant sticks in flour, then in beaten eggs, and then coat with bread crumb mixture. Place on a plate and let rest for 5-6 minutes.

4

Preheat an air fryer to 370 degrees F.

5

Place eggplant sticks in basket, making sure they are not touching; cook in batches if necessary.

6

Cook in the preheated air fryer for 9 minutes. Shake basket and continue cooking to desired crispiness, an additional 4 to 6 minutes.

Nutrition
Per Serving: 180 calories; protein 9.6g; carbohydrates 25.4g; fat 5.1g; cholesterol 97.6mg; sodium 960mg.

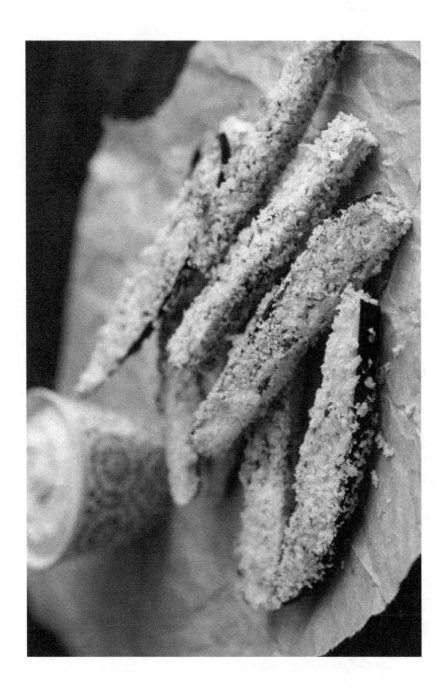

Tuna Sandwich

Prep:

15 mins

Total:

15 mins

Servings:

2

Yield:

2 servings

Ingredients

1 (5 ounce) can tuna, drained

¼ cup mayonnaise

1 tablespoon chopped dill pickles

2 leaves lettuce

2 slices Swiss cheese

1 ½ teaspoons cream-style horseradish sauce

4 slices bread

2 thin slices red onion

2 slices tomato

Directions

1

Combine the drained tuna, mayonnaise, horseradish sauce, and pickles in a small bowl until evenly mixed. Place a slice of Swiss cheese onto 2 slices of bread, and top with a leaf of lettuce. Spread the tuna mixture onto the lettuce leaves. Top with the tomato and red onion slices, and finish with the remaining slices of bread.

Nutrition

Per Serving: 529 calories; protein 28.3g; carbohydrates 30.2g; fat 32.7g; cholesterol 56.9mg; sodium 645.3mg.

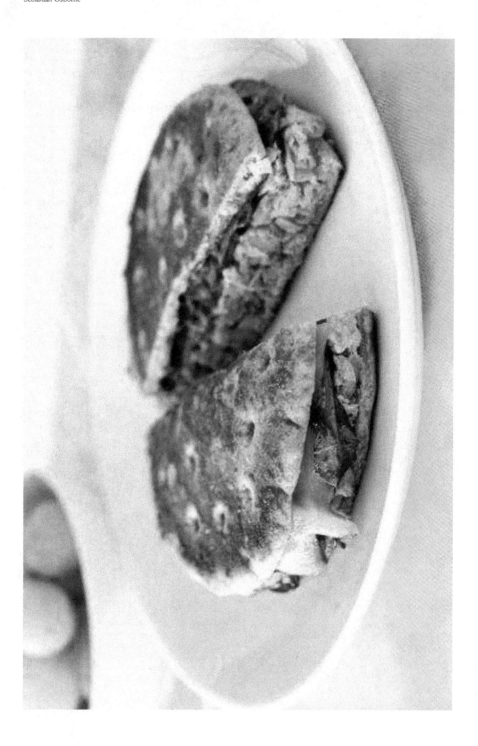

Lasagna

Prep:

30 mins

Cook:

30 mins

Total:

1 hr

Servings:

8

Yield:

1 9x13 inch pan

Ingredients

1 (16 ounce) package lasagna noodles
½ pound shredded Cheddar cheese
1 pound lean ground beef
1 (16 ounce) jar spaghetti sauce
1 clove garlic, minced
½ pound shredded mozzarella cheese
salt and pepper to taste
1 pint ricotta cheese

Directions

1

Bring a large pot of lightly salted water to a boil. Add pasta and cook for 8 to 10 minutes or until al dente; drain.

2

Preheat oven to 350 degrees F. In a large skillet over medium-high heat, brown beef and season with salt and pepper; drain. Stir in spaghetti sauce and garlic and simmer 5 minutes.

3

In a medium bowl, combine mozzarella, Cheddar and ricotta; stir well. In 9x13 inch pan, alternate layers of noodles, meat mixture and cheese mixture until pan is filled.

4

Bake in preheated oven for 30 minutes, or until cheese is melted and bubbly.

Nutrition

Per Serving: 643 calories; protein 41.3g; carbohydrates 53.4g; fat 29.3g; cholesterol 108.3mg; sodium 707.3mg.

Farfalle Festival

Prep:

20 mins

Cook:

20 mins

Total:

40 mins

Servings:

2

Yield:

2 servings

Ingredients

10 ounces farfalle (bow tie) pasta

4 slices bacon, diced

1 tablespoon butter

1 teaspoon chopped garlic

¼ cup diced Roma tomatoes

1 cooked chicken breast, thinly sliced

2 tablespoons diced red onion

1 pinch ground black pepper

1 pinch garlic salt

2 tablespoons heavy cream

2 tablespoons grated Asiago cheese

1 pinch salt

⅓ cup Alfredo sauce

Directions

1

Fill a large pot with lightly salted water and bring to a rolling boil over high heat. Stir in the bow tie pasta and return to a boil. Cook, uncovered, stirring occasionally, until the pasta is cooked through but still firm to the bite, about 12 minutes. Drain.

2

Meanwhile, cook the bacon in a skillet over medium heat until nearly crisp, about 5 minutes. Remove the bacon and wipe out the skillet with a paper towel.

3

Melt the butter in the same skillet over medium heat. Return the bacon to the skillet, and stir in the red onion, garlic, Roma tomatoes, chicken, black pepper, garlic salt, and salt. Cook and stir until the bacon is crisp and onions are translucent. Stir in the cream and Asiago cheese, and cook until the liquid is reduced by half, about 3 minutes.

4

Stir in the Alfredo sauce and the cooked pasta. Remove from heat, and allow to cool slightly before serving.

Nutrition

Per Serving: 928 calories; protein 43.1g; carbohydrates 107.2g; fat 37.6g; cholesterol 114.7mg; sodium 1150.1mg.

Fattoush

Prep:

1 hr

Total:

1 hr

Servings:

6

Yield:

6 servings

Ingredients

6 lettuce leaves, chopped

3 cabbage leaves, chopped

1 medium cucumber, diced

1 red bell pepper, minced

1 carrot, shredded

¼ cup sweet corn kernels

2 small radishes, minced

1 large tomato, finely diced

1 small onion, sliced thin

¼ cup pomegranate syrup

12 sprigs parsley, minced

12 mint leaves, minced

2 large cloves garlic, crushed

¼ cup olive oil

Directions

1

Toss together the lettuce, cabbage, radish, cucumber, red bell pepper, carrot, corn, tomato, onion, garlic, parsley, mint, olive oil, pomegranate seeds, and pomegranate syrup in a large bowl.

2

Heat oil in a deep-fryer or saucepan to 350 degrees F . Fry the pita breads until golden in color. Remove to cool on paper towels. Crush the bread into small pieces; sprinkle over the salad.

Nutrition

Per Serving: 257 calories; protein 4.8g; carbohydrates 23.5g; fat 17.3g; sodium 137.6mg.

Dill Gazpacho

Prep:

25 mins

Additional:

1 hr

Total:

1 hr 25 mins

Servings:

6

Yield:

6 servings

Ingredients

6 medium ripe tomatoes, finely chopped
1 onion, finely chopped
1 green bell pepper, finely chopped
jalapeno pepper, seeded and minced
1 large lemon, juiced
2 cucumbers, peeled and finely chopped
1 tablespoon balsamic vinegar
2 teaspoons olive oil
1 teaspoon kosher salt
¼ cup chopped fresh dill
½ teaspoon ground black pepper

Directions

1

In a large bowl, stir together tomatoes, cucumber, onion, bell pepper, and jalapeno pepper. Season with lemon juice, balsamic vinegar, olive oil, salt and pepper.

2

In a blender or food processor, puree half of the mixture until smooth. Return to bowl, stir in dill and mix well. Cover and chill for at least one hour before serving.

Nutrition

Per Serving: 58 calories; protein 2g; carbohydrates 10.9g; fat 2g; sodium 330.3mg.

CHAPTER 4: SNACK & APPETIZER

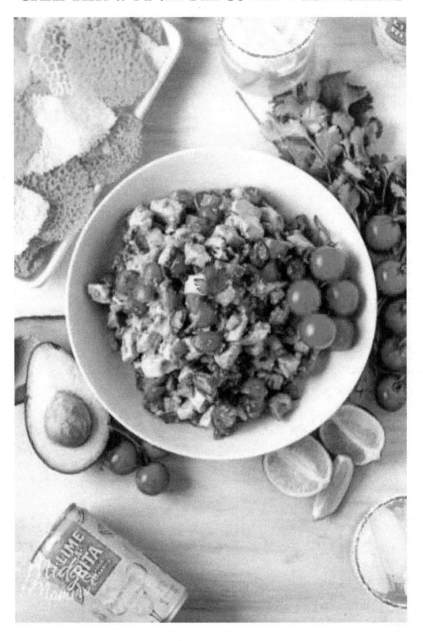

Avocado Dip

Prep:

30 mins

Cook:

13 mins

Total:

43 mins

Servings:

3

Yield:

3 servings

Ingredients

2 Hass avocado, peeled and pitted

2 green plantains, peeled and sliced into fifths

1 tablespoon lemon juice

¼ teaspoon salt

1 clove garlic, minced

vegetable oil for frying

1 tablespoon mayonnaise

Directions

1

Combine avocados, lemon juice, mayonnaise, and salt together in a bowl; sprinkle in garlic. Mash using a potato masher until dip is creamy.

2

Heat oil in a deep-fryer or large saucepan to 350 degrees F. Drizzle about 1 teaspoon oil onto a clean work surface and the bottom of a coffee cup.

3

Fry the plantains in the hot oil until golden brown, 8 to 10 minutes. Remove from fryer and place on the work surface; flatten with the bottom of the coffee cup. Re-fry until browned and tender, about 5 minutes. Place on a paper towel-covered plate; sprinkle with salt. Serve plantains alongside the dip.

Nutrition

Per Serving: 830 calories; protein 1.7g; carbohydrates 39g; fat 77.4g; cholesterol 1.7mg; sodium 224.9mg.

Baba Ghanoush

Prep:

5 mins

Cook:

40 mins

Additional:

3 hrs

Total:

3 hrs 45 mins

Servings:

12

Yield:

1 1/2 cups

Ingredients

1 eggplant

¼ cup lemon juice

2 cloves garlic, minced

salt and pepper to taste

1 ½ tablespoons olive oil

¼ cup tahini

2 tablespoons sesame seeds

Directions

1

Preheat oven to 400 degrees F. Lightly grease a baking sheet.

2

Place eggplant on baking sheet, and make holes in the skin with a fork. Roast it for 30 to 40 minutes, turning occasionally, or until soft. Remove from oven, and place into a large bowl of cold water. Remove from water, and peel skin off.

3

Place eggplant, lemon juice, tahini, sesame seeds, and garlic in an electric blender, and puree. Season with salt and pepper to taste. Transfer eggplant mixture to a medium size mixing bowl, and slowly mix in olive oil. Refrigerate for 3 hours before serving.

Nutrition

Per Serving: 66 calories; protein 1.6g; carbohydrates 4.6g; fat 5.2g; sodium 7mg.

Stromboli Bites

Prep:

15 mins

Cook:

45 mins

Additional:

11 hrs

Total:

12 hrs

Servings:

10

Yield:

10 servings

Ingredients

½ pound Italian sausage

⅓ cup cornmeal

1 (1 pound) loaf frozen bread dough

6 slices pepperoni sausage

1 tablespoon yellow mustard

1 tablespoon prepared Dijon-style mustard

5 slices cooked ham

6 slices salami

4 slices provolone cheese

4 slices processed American cheese

1 teaspoon dried oregano

1 teaspoon dried basil

Directions

1

Allow frozen bread dough to thaw approximately 8 hours, or overnight, in the refrigerator. Place dough in a large, lightly greased bowl. Place bowl in a warm location, and allow dough to rise until doubled (2 to 3 hours). Punch down dough.

2

Place Italian sausage in a large, deep skillet. Cook over medium high heat until evenly brown. Drain and set aside.

3

Preheat oven to 325 degrees F. Lightly grease a large baking sheet.

4

Roll dough into an approximately 10x14 inch rectangle on the baking sheet. Spread with yellow mustard and prepared Dijon-style mustard. Line center with cooked Italian sausage, ham, pepperoni sausage, salami, provolone cheese and American cheese. Sprinkle with oregano and basil.

5

Fold edges of dough over the fillings and pinch together. Tuck and pinch ends. Sprinkle with cornmeal, and flip so the seam side is down.

6

Bake in the preheated oven 45 minutes, or until a deep golden brown. Cool 10 minutes before cutting into bite-sized slices.

Nutrition

Per Serving: 344 calories; protein 18.8g; carbohydrates 16g; fat 23g; cholesterol 61.9mg; sodium 1132.6mg.

Seeds Bars

Prep:

20 mins

Cook:

20 mins

Total:

40 mins

Servings:

24

Yield:

24 servings

Ingredients

4 cups old-fashioned rolled oats

1 cup brown sugar, packed

1 cup wheat germ

2 cups whole wheat flour

2 eggs, beaten

1 cup honey

1 cup canola oil

2 teaspoons vanilla extract

1 teaspoon cinnamon

½ cup semi-sweet chocolate chips

1 teaspoon salt

½ cup flax seeds

½ cup sesame seeds

½ cup sunflower seeds

Directions

1

Preheat oven to 350 degrees F. Lightly grease a 9x14 inch ovenproof baking dish.

2

Mix the rolled oats, brown sugar, wheat germ, cinnamon, and flour together in a large bowl. In a separate bowl, whisk together the eggs, honey, canola oil, vanilla, and salt until evenly blended., and stir into the oat mixture. Stir in the flax seeds, sesame seeds, sunflower seeds, and chocolate chips. Use your hands to mix the **Ingredients**, and press the mixture into the prepared pan.

3

Bake in preheated oven until the edges are golden brown, 20 to 25 minutes. Cool completely in the baking dish before cutting into 2 inch bars.

Nutrition

Per Serving: 321 calories; protein 6.1g; carbohydrates 43.5g; fat 15.2g; cholesterol 15.5mg; sodium 109.5mg.

Yogurt Protein Bowl

Prep:

5 mins

Total:

5 mins

Servings:

1

Yield:

1 serving

Ingredients

¼ cup Greek yogurt

½ chocolate protein bar, cut into small pieces

5 fresh strawberries, sliced

1 tablespoon peanut butter

Directions

1

Combine Greek yogurt and peanut butter in a bowl and whip together until smooth. Top with protein bar pieces and strawberries.

Nutrition

Per Serving: 305 calories; protein 12.9g; carbohydrates 34.6g; fat 14g; cholesterol 11.3mg; sodium 140.5mg.

CHAPTER 5: SMOOTHIES & DRINKS RECIPES

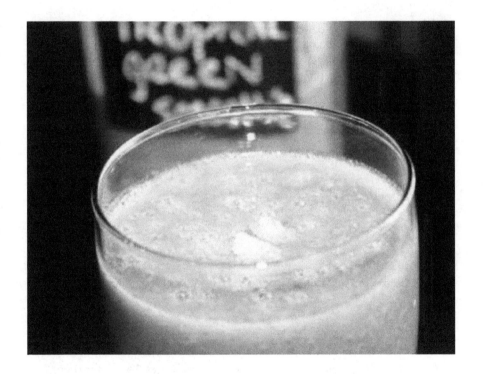

Green Delight

Prep:

5 mins

Total:

5 mins

Servings:

1

Yield:

1 glass

Ingredients

½ cup frozen blueberries

2 cups iced green tea

4 frozen strawberries

Directions

1

Place the blueberries and strawberries in the bottom of a tall glass. Pour the green tea over the berries.

Nutrition

Per Serving: 59 calories; protein 0.5g; carbohydrates 14.7g; fat 0.6g; sodium 15.8mg.

Coconut Smoothie

Prep:

10 mins

Total:

10 mins

Servings:

2

Yield:

2 smoothies

Ingredients

2 bananas

1 cup water

⅓ cup coconut milk

1 tablespoon almond butter

1 tablespoon moringa powder

1 cup sliced frozen peaches

Directions

1

Layer bananas, peaches, coconut milk, moringa powder, and almond butter in a blender; add water. Blend mixture until very smooth, at least 1 minute.

Nutrition

Per Serving: 252 calories; protein 4g; carbohydrates 34.7g; fat 13.2g; sodium 48.2mg

Carrot Juice

Prep:

10 mins

Total:

10 mins

Servings:

1

Yield:

1 float

Ingredients

2 large carrots

¼ cup vanilla ice cream

Directions

1

Wash the carrots and trim the tops off, then juice using a juice machine. Pour the carrot juice over the ice cream to serve.

Nutrition

Per Serving: 125 calories; protein 2.5g; carbohydrates 21.6g; fat 4g; cholesterol 14.5mg; sodium 125.8mg.

Cucumber Smoothie

Prep:

10 mins

Total:

10 mins

Servings:

1

Yield:

1 smoothie

Ingredients

1 frozen banana, cut into chunks

2 tablespoons blueberry preserves

¾ cup buttermilk

¼ cup coconut water

½ cucumber - peeled, seeded, and cut into chunks

Directions

1

Blend banana, cucumber, buttermilk, coconut water, and blueberry preserves together in a blender until smooth.

Nutrition

Per Serving: 252 calories; protein 8.4g; carbohydrates 53.5g; fat 2.3g; cholesterol 7.3mg; sodium 264.1mg.

CHAPTER 6: DESSERTS

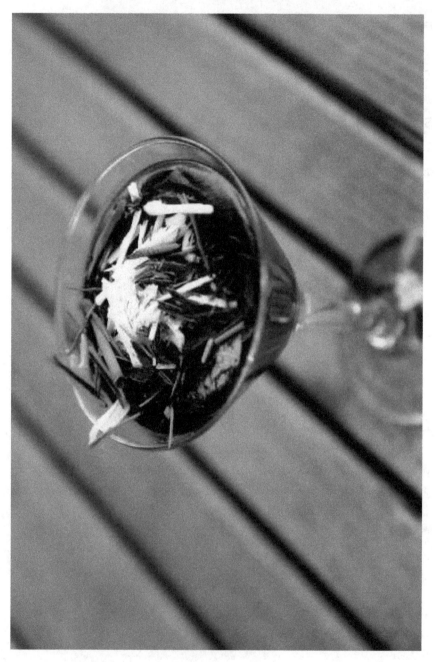

Avocado Pudding

Prep:

5 mins

Additional:

1 hr

Total:

1 hr 5 mins

Servings:

1

Yield:

1 serving

Ingredients

1 ripe avocado

2 packets stevia sugar substitute (such as Truvia®)

⅓ cup heavy cream

1 pinch salt

½ teaspoon vanilla extract

Directions

1

Combine avocado, cream, sweetener, vanilla extract, and salt in a blender; blend until smooth. Chill for 1 hour.

Nutrition

Per Serving: 604 calories; protein 5.6g; carbohydrates 21.6g; fat 58.8g; cholesterol 108.7mg; sodium 199.4mg.

Pomegranate Granita

Prep:

10 mins

Total:

10 mins

Servings:

1

Yield:

1 cocktail

Ingredients

1 cup ice
2 teaspoons white sugar
1 (1.5 fluid ounce) jigger Cointreau or other orange liqueur
2 fluid ounces pomegranate syrup
1 orange slice
½ (1.5 fluid ounce) jigger white rum

Directions

1

Place the ice, Cointreau, rum, and pomegranate syrup into a blender, blend until smooth. Moisten the rim of a tumbler with the cut edge of the orange slice, and dip the glass into the sugar to line the rim. Pour the granita into the glass, and garnish with the orange slice to serve.

Nutrition

Per Serving: 387 calories; protein 0g; carbohydrates 66.4g; fat 0.1g; cholesterol 0mg; sodium 10.4mg.

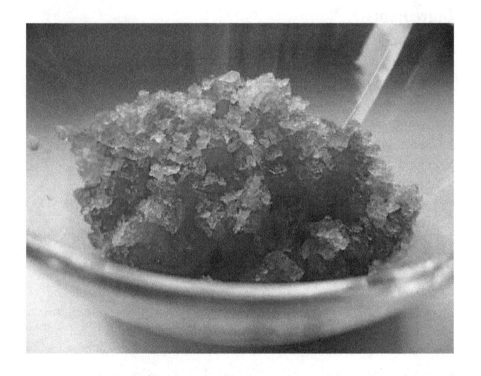

Rhubarb Pie

Servings:

8

Yield:

1 - 9 inch pie

Ingredients

3 ½ cups diced rhubarb
½ cup white sugar
1 recipe pastry for a 9 inch single crust pie
¼ cup butter
1 tablespoon all-purpose flour
½ cup packed brown sugar
½ cup all-purpose flour
½ cup crushed cornflakes cereal

Directions

1

Combine rhubarb, 1 tablespoon flour and white sugar. Mix well and place in pie shell.

2

Melt the butter or margarine and mix with 1/2 cup brown sugar, crushed corn flakes and 1/2 cup flour. Mix in a bowl and pat down on top of pie. Bake in oven at 350 degrees F for about 40 minutes. Turn off oven and leave the pie in the oven for another hour. Serve warm.

Nutrition

Per Serving: 315 calories; protein 3g; carbohydrates 46.9g; fat 13.4g; cholesterol 15.3mg; sodium 176.6mg

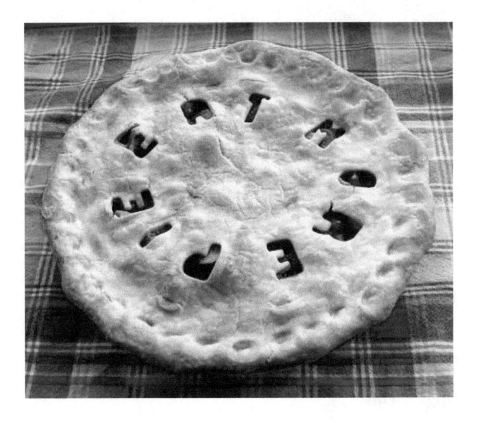

Carrot Cake

Prep:

30 mins

Cook:

55 mins

Additional:

35 mins

Total:

2 hrs

Servings:

15

Yield:

15 to 18 servings

Ingredients

2 cups white sugar

¾ cup buttermilk

¾ cup vegetable oil

1 teaspoon vanilla extract

3 eggs

1 teaspoon vanilla extract

1 (15 ounce) can crushed pineapple, drained

2 cups grated carrots

1 cup flaked coconut

2 cups all-purpose flour

2 teaspoons baking soda

2 teaspoons ground cinnamon

1 cup chopped walnuts

½ cup butter

1 ½ teaspoons salt

1 (8 ounce) package cream cheese

4 cups confectioners' sugar

Directions

1

Preheat oven to 350 degrees F. Grease a 9x13 inch baking pan. Set aside.

2

In a large bowl, mix together sugar, oil, eggs, vanilla, and buttermilk. Stir in carrots, coconut, vanilla, and pineapple. In a separate bowl, combine flour, baking soda, cinnamon, and salt; gently stir into carrot mixture. Stir in chopped nuts. Spread batter into prepared pan.

3

Bake for 55 minutes or until toothpick inserted into cake comes out clean. Remove from oven, and set aside to cool.

4

In a medium mixing bowl, combine butter or margarine, cream cheese, vanilla, and confectioners sugar. Blend until creamy. Frost cake while still in the pan.

Nutrition

Per Serving: 616 calories; protein 6.2g; carbohydrates 83.5g; fat 30.2g; cholesterol 70.4mg; sodium 540.4mg

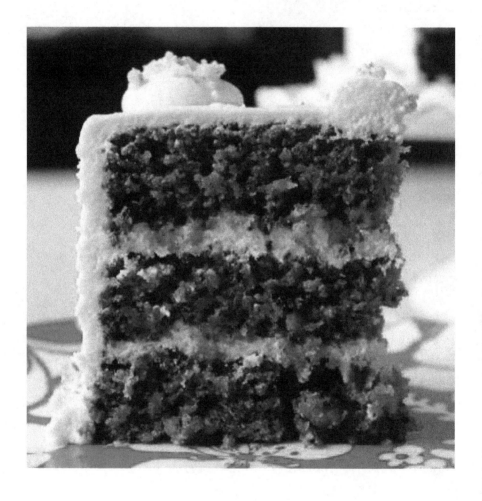

Mango Crumble

Prep:

20 mins

Cook:

20 mins

Total:

40 mins

Servings:

4

Yield:

4 servings

Ingredients

¾ cup all-purpose flour

2 teaspoons ground cinnamon

⅓ cup brown sugar

6 tablespoons cold butter

⅔ cup rolled oats

½ teaspoon ground nutmeg

2 passion fruit, pulp removed

1 tablespoon lime juice

1 pinch ground cinnamon

2 ripe mangoes - peeled, pitted, and cubed

Directions

1

Preheat an oven to 350 degrees F. Grease an 8x8 inch baking dish.

2

Mix the flour and brown sugar in a bowl, and cut the butter into the flour-sugar mixture with a pastry cutter or two table knives until the mixture resembles coarse cornmeal. Add the oats, cinnamon, and nutmeg, and stir well.

3

Place the cubed mango on the bottom of the greased baking dish, and spoon the passion fruit pulp over the mango. Stir to mix and evenly distribute the fruit in the dish. Drizzle lime juice over the fruit. Sprinkle the fruit with the oats topping, making sure it is fully covered. Sprinkle a little extra cinnamon over the top.

4

Bake in the preheated oven until the top has browned and the fruit is tender, about 20 minutes.

Nutrition

Per Serving: 423 calories; protein 5.1g; carbohydrates 61.5g; fat 18.8g; cholesterol 45.8mg; sodium 133.4mg.

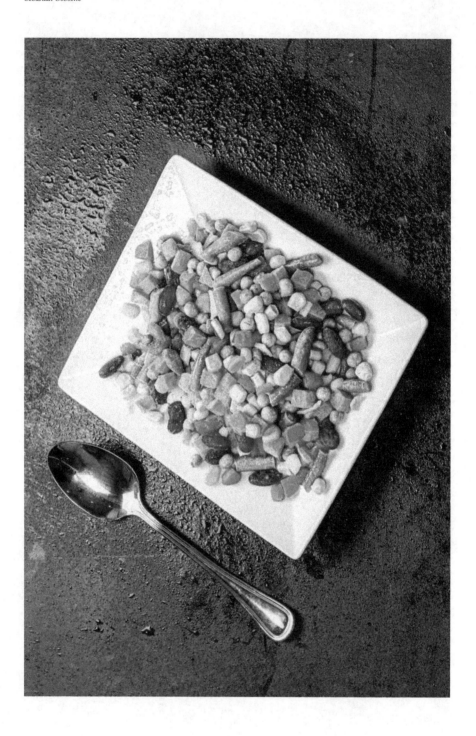

CPSIA information can be obtained
at www.ICGtesting.com
Printed in the USA
BVHW090441290421
605864BV00024B/514